Coronary Caring Without Tears

CW01091444

Coronary Caring Without Tears

Positive Help
for Heart Attack Sufferers
and their Families

Lysbeth Rose

ANGUS
& ROBERTSON
PUBLISHERS

AUGUS & ROBERTSON PUBLISHERS

Unit 4, Eden Park, 31 Waterloo Road,
North Ryde, NSW, Australia 2113, and
16 Golden Square, London W1R 4BN, United Kingdom

First published in Australia by Angus & Robertson Publishers in 1985
First published in the United Kingdom by Angus & Robertson (UK) Ltd in 1985

Copyright © Lysbeth Rose 1985

National Library of Australia
Cataloguing-in-publication data.

Rose, Lysbeth.
    Coronary caring without tears.

    ISBN 0 207 15081 8.

    1. Cardiacs—Rehabilitation. I. Rose, Lysbeth.
    Coronary wife. II. Title. III. Title: Coronary wife.

616.1'23

Typeset in 12 pt Baskerville by Graphicraft Typesetters
Printed in Great Britain by
Richard Clay (The Chaucer Press) Ltd,
Bungay, Suffolk

To S.J.M.G. and J.G.R.
*with affection and gratitude
for all their care and kindness*

Contents

Foreword

There is a great need for a book such as this to help the families of coronary sufferers. This man's story, written in an easily read, positive-thinking way by his wife, gives much practical assistance.

The book describes the ten-year progression of her husband's illness, from the first heart attack through to slowly developing angina, which becomes crippling and is then cured by coronary-artery bypass surgery. There are descriptions of the modern tests used to assess the function of the heart and, of course, of the operation and why it is necessary. The information on heart attack risk factors should be heeded by all, whether they have heart disease or not.

The story is in a sense commonplace—thousands of Australians have bypass surgery and recover each year. Commonplace until the need for the operation strikes a family member or close friend. That is when this book with its very human account will be a helpful guide and a reassuring friend, particularly the section on rehabilitation after the operation. This phase, once control by professionals has passed, involves patient and family (in this case, wife) being suddenly on their own and having tremendous readjustments to make. Even if only for this section, the book should be recommended reading for all in the same situation. It

is a valuable account of angina and coronary-artery
bypass surgery.

R. L. Hodge
MB, BS, MD, FRACP
Director,
National Heart
Foundation of Australia

Preface

I have written this book to help other families cope with some of the everyday problems that occur when a normally active person is suddenly stricken by a coronary occlusion or has to undergo coronary-artery bypass surgery.

It is a completely factual account of my own experiences and, to the best of my knowledge, the accounts of what happened to others are also true, although for obvious reasons the names used throughout are fictitious. As no two cases are exactly the same, a patient's family should not hesitate to ask the doctor just how much and what the patient can do as he or she progressively improves.

In every case the doctor's thorough knowledge of the patient will help effect more rapid progress. The problems and worries that this book describes are all of interest to the doctor and discussion of them can go a long way towards alleviating a family's stress. Should you have a problem that is not covered in this book, don't ask well-meaning friends for advice; ask your doctor.

My thanks go to the many people and organisations who willingly supplied information, and especially to specialists in various fields at the Royal Prince Alfred Hospital, Sydney, and the National Heart Foundation;

to Mr Douglas Baird, Chairman of the Cardiac
Surgery Committee of the National Heart Foundation
of Australia and to Dr Robert Hodge, Director of the
National Heart Foundation of Australia, for assistance
with this book; and to my husband for allowing his
story to be told.

L.R.

Introduction

Why is the heart so important?

Many people are vague about the functions and action of the heart. They know that it pumps blood around the body and that if it stops the owner will die, and they have read much in recent years about the more spectacular types of heart surgery. The heart is a more perfect pump than any devised by humankind. Over seventy times a minute for, on an average, seventy years it pumps blood into the circulatory system, usually without the need for any maintenance or running repairs.

Our blood is our life-line. It transports all over the body those substances our cells need in order to live and function properly, and it removes waste products and gases from the cells. Oxygen absorbed from the air breathed into the lungs is carried by the blood to the cells, and when this is used by the cells the blood carries the carbon dioxide that results back to the lungs to be exhaled. Food digested in the alimentary canal and broken down to usable and absorbable substances is also carried by the blood to the cells; after the cells have used what they require, the blood carries the waste products to the kidneys for elimination.

Fresh blood is conveyed around the body by the arteries. Because this blood contains oxygen it is bright red. Used blood, which is darker and more blue in colour, returns to the heart through the veins. To carry out their functions arteries and veins divide and subdivide—as a main road divides into subsidiary roads until finally lanes and driveways to homes are reached—until they have become the tiny capillaries that ooze blood when you prick your finger. The blood from the arteries reaches the cells by way of the capillaries, and then by way of other capillaries blood returns to the veins.

The heart is made up of a special type of muscle and is divided into two pairs of chambers, each pair consisting of a collecting chamber called the auricle and a pumping chamber called the ventricle. A partition down the centre separates the left auricle and ventricle from the right auricle and ventricle. Fresh, oxygenated blood from the lungs enters the heart at the left auricle, passes through a valve into the left ventricle, and from here is pumped around the body at the rate of about six litres a minute. Used blood returns to the heart at the right auricle, passes into the right ventricle, and is then pumped to the lungs, where the cycle begins again. This continuous pumping from the heart, around the body, and back to the lungs is referred to as the circulation of the blood.

The heart has its own blood supply, called the coronary circulation. As in the rest of the body, large arteries, smaller arteries, and capillaries bring fresh blood to its muscle cells, and veins remove the waste products. If one of these coronary arteries becomes partially blocked or narrowed the blood supply to the heart cells is greatly reduced. Chest pains (angina) may result. A heart attack—a coronary occlusion or

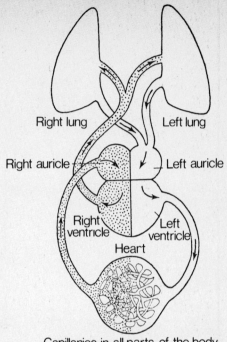

Right lung

Left lung

Right auricle

Left auricle

Right ventricle

Left ventricle

Heart

Capillaries in all parts of the body

Diagram showing the circulation of the blood.

coronary thrombosis—occurs when one of these diseased coronary arteries is suddenly blocked by a clot of blood. The heart muscle is then damaged. The severity of the coronary and thus the length of the period before normal life can be resumed depend upon the size and importance of the coronary artery involved, and the length of time before treatment is commenced.

A coronary nearly always occurs suddenly, so it is often dramatic for the patient and his or her relatives.

PART I:
THE CORONARY

CHAPTER 1

Personal Drama

The doctor told me to go home and take a sleeping tablet. The physical examination, electrocardiograph, X-rays, and preliminary tests were all finished for the night. My husband's coronary was apparently a mild one. There was practically no danger of his succumbing to it; he was comparatively young—in his late forties. I should get a good night's rest.

My husband smiled wanly. "I'll be all right," he said. "The pain has gone now. Don't you worry, darling."

Some hope!

It was after 10 p.m. when, wrung out, I put the car in the garage. Our nineteen-year-old son, alerted by a friend, had returned from a party. He threw open the door for me.

"Is Dad all right, Mum? What happened?"

My husband is a surgeon, and for years his greatest relaxation has been sailing. When he bought his first boat, an ancient, open eighteen-footer, gaff-rigged and with a centreboard, the children and I, and various friends, accompanied him every weekend. I was always terrified. However, I learnt a little about sailing, and he became really keen. He graduated to racing. In newer, faster, and larger boats he raced with a crew of enthusiastic males on Saturdays, and, weather permitting, we had picnic days on Sundays.

Of course he used to hope that he would some day have his dream boat, and one November "she" became available, at a price we could afford. Oldish, not the fastest boat in the world, but equipped with bunks, stove, sink, and toilet, it meant that we would be able to have holidays on board — really "get away from it all". And he could still race with the Third Division.

Early in December he and some friends sailed out of Sydney Harbour and up the coast to Pittwater. A friend who had a mooring there wanted to bring his boat to Port Jackson, so we had arranged to swap moorings. We had five glorious days and nights on board just before Christmas, returned to Sydney by car for a few days, and then set off for another five days over the New Year period — just the two of us.

We took an Esky full of cooked food, a carton of provisions, clothes, and reading matter, carried them down the two hundred metres through our friend's property to the beach, loaded them in the dinghy, and rowed out to the boat, anchored about a hundred metres off shore. It was about 5 p.m. At the next mooring a retired doctor we knew was pottering about on his boat. We waved, and began stowing the gear. My husband pumped out the bilge down below while I pushed the sails on deck. I was putting up the flag when he came up from the cabin, sweating and an awful colour.

"Are you all right?" I asked in alarm.

"I feel peculiar. I think I'll rest a bit," he said, and stretched out in the cockpit. I fished out some cushions.

4

"Shall I call over Dr Smith?" I said. "He's still there."

"No. Don't fuss. It was a bit hot down below, that's all. I'll be all right."

We had the radio tuned to the last of the cricket test match, so we sat there listening. My husband still looked ill. He drank some brandy, which seemed to have little effect. Trying not to show my concern, I once again suggested calling the doctor on the next boat, but he would not hear of it.

By this time he was complaining of some pain and was obviously very uncomfortable. I was beginning to be alarmed, although he still insisted it was nothing and that it would pass. The only pain-killer we had in the first aid kit was some Panadol, but that did not help him much either. And Dr Smith had rowed ashore.

The cricket finished at 6 p.m. and he said, "Darling, I'm sorry, but I do feel ill. We'll have to go home." I knew then that he must be really bad, because he had been so looking forward to this little holiday.

"You just stay there for a minute," I said as I began putting the sails away, wondering all the while how I—only about fifty-five kilograms—would get him—about ninety-six kilograms—into the dinghy, and after that ashore and up to the car.

Some men had been water skiing in the bay, and they were at that time preparing to go home and were within hailing distance. They came alongside, took in the situation, and were wonderful. After almost carrying my husband into their speedboat (with padded seats!), one of them helped me put things away and load on to their boat the food and gear we could not leave aboard, and they towed the dinghy to the beach.

"Where's your car?" one asked. When I explained about the longish walk uphill to the road, he told me they lived at the other end of the beach within a few yards of the road; it would be better if I drove the car there so my husband would not have so far to walk. One of them stowed the dinghy and then they both set off in the speedboat taking my husband and the gear.

Having told our friend (the husband was in town) what had happened, I asked her to try to contact our son who, I knew, had planned to go out for the evening. I thought perhaps she could catch him at home before he left. Then I drove to where our rescuers lived. Those men were absolutely marvellous; they helped my husband to the car and loaded everything into the boot for me. And so we set off for home. I must confess I feared that he might not last the distance. Although the temperature was about 26°C he wore his thick, navy-type polo-neck sweater, the car rug was over him, and still he asked for the heaters to be turned on. I was very frightened; never do I want to live through a drive like that again.

In most of the districts we passed through there was at least one doctor he knew or who would have known him, but no matter how often I suggested stopping he kept saying no, no, he just wanted to get home. I thought it best not to agitate him by insisting. I had felt his pulse earlier, and it was strong and seemed to me to be even. At Mosman, where there was a good friend in practice, he still refused to allow me to stop. But when we were almost home he suddenly said,

6

"Don't go home. Drive straight to John's." John is a physician attached to Royal Prince Alfred Hospital and lives near us.

Still in my shorts I rushed in. It was about 8 p.m. John had just arrived home from hospital, and he had not yet had his dinner. He hurried out to the car, examined my husband quickly, gave him some pain-killer, and arranged for his immediate admission to Royal Prince Alfred Hospital.

"I think he has had a slight coronary," he said, "but apart from the distress caused by the chest pain, which should ease shortly, his condition is quite good. I'll come to the hospital with you."

I hurriedly changed into something more present-able and asked John's daughter to try to contact our son at his friend's home, to tell him we were going straight to the hospital.

At the hospital we were met by men with a trolley. The necessary tests were carried out immediately, and I waited, trying to appear composed.

No matter where or when a person has a coronary it is dramatic—for the person, for the partner, for the family. In the case of the man I shall call Alec the attack was mild enough and occurred in the early hours of the morning, but it happened to be the day his only son began the Higher School Certificate examina-tions. The doctor was spirited in while the boy was in the shower, and he examined the patient behind the closed bedroom door while the wife, pretending that Father was sleeping in after having had a very late night, gave the boy breakfast and sent him off to school unaware of what had happened. It might be like Jim's attack, when he was racing a small boat, with his twelve-year-old daughter acting as for'ard hand, and she had to bring him back to the beach where, fortunately, there was plenty of help. Or it might be at the theatre or a concert, or during a large official dinner, or on the golf course or bowling green.

"Go home and take a sleeping tablet and don't worry," they tell you. The partner still has to relive the drama in telling the immediate family what has happened. If the children are young the partner's own great fears have to be hidden, not only for their loved one's immediate safety, but also for the future. And when, next day, they go to the hospital, they have to try to be bright and cheerful so as not to worry the patient.

CHAPTER 2

But Why?

So after I had told my son the story, we had a cup of tea and unloaded the car. Sadly and wearily I put things back into the refrigerator; so much for that little holiday. But — when were we likely to have another few days away on the boat? What about the boat? Would he ever be able to sail it again? It was ironic that having just acquired his dream boat after all the years of wishing, it looked as though he would not be able to enjoy it. I began remembering things that were still on board and that should have come home — blankets, portable radio, and the like. My son said he would fetch them, and he would put on the cover and make sure everything was all right at the weekend.

I took a sleeping tablet, but as I climbed alone into bed the implications began to hit me.

We were married during the war, and the years of separation and my anxieties when he was in combat zones probably helped bind us more closely together. Although we have both kept our own interests and they have not always coincided, we have always had the greatest pleasure from doing things together. Through life we have shared a number of great sorrows as well as great joys, and always he has been the most important person in my life.

He is very dedicated to his profession. When our two children were small we all set off for England for about two years (at our own expense; there were few grants given in those days) so that he could gain further training and experience. We shall always remember those years. During one summer we took a caravan for three months. We went to Scotland for a fortnight first, to get used to it without having to cope with foreign languages and driving on the other side of the road, and then we went to Europe and Scandinavia. We camped by fjords in Norway, in pine forests in Sweden, in olive groves in Italy, and in the central squares of small towns in France. Our daughter (then aged seven) learnt to count to ten in every language, and our son (who was five) to ask for ice-cream and toilets. They also learnt that children enjoy the same games everywhere. When we were in camping areas and other children were about, someone would produce a ball or a skipping-rope, and immediately a game would commence, each child chattering in his own language and all somehow understanding.

On our return to Sydney my husband made the great decision to specialise in a branch of surgery. Five years later he went to America and England to see recent advances in his speciality, and we spent two or three weeks on holiday in Europe, visiting places we had not seen when we were living there.

When our daughter had completed her university course she, like so many of her friends, took off for Europe as soon as she had saved some money. So on our last trip overseas, in 1968, when he had finished six weeks of pretty solid professional work in America, we flew to Paris where she joined us, and for the next three months she travelled with us. There were two big international conferences—one in England and one in Greece—during this period, and we had many friends to see. We took two or three weeks' holiday, hiring a car in Copenhagen and driving leisurely to Rome, and after the second conference, in Athens, we again had a few days' relaxation—on one of the Greek islands —before going to Israel where my husband had been asked to lecture. Our daughter stayed there and we came home via Singapore, where there was a little more work lecturing and helping to cement ties in medicine between Australia and South-East Asia.

As I lay in bed that night I kept thinking, "Was it the trip that put too much strain on him?" We had been back about three months. I had insisted on weekends of rest and relaxation during the very hectic stay in America, where they start work at 7 a.m. and often there are meetings and lectures in the evenings as well. I came to the conclusion that we could not blame the trip.

So why? Why did my husband, who was in the prime of life, and hardly ever ill apart from an annual attack of laryngitis—he didn't even suffer from headaches—why did he suddenly, during a quiet period of the year, suffer a coronary?

I wondered about our social life. We enjoy going out. We love the theatre, concerts, and ballet, and visiting friends. Had life been too hectic? Was it too much to expect a man who worked hard all day to go out in the evenings? And yet, the quality of life depends on more than meals, work and sleep. Through the years he had developed a certain amount of resistance:

he enjoys a game of cards, but refused to go to large card parties; he supports many charities, but would only attend charity "dos" if it was something to which I particularly wanted to go. I thought back and could not see that our social activities would have caused this attack.

Work? Well, he worked extremely hard; operations sometimes lasted four or five hours. Of course we did not go out during the evening following such a day. Emergency night calls? Yes, especially during the weeks he was honorary surgeon for hospital admissions; sometimes he would get only a few hours' sleep. If we had tickets for a concert or the theatre the next night and he was tired, I would go with a friend.

While there was no single cause, all these things added up. After returning from overseas there had been a great build-up of work to be coped with, and unfortunately there had been a certain amount of chaos in his department caused by the premature resignation of one of his assistants. He came home to extra operating, no staff work done, and a rather discontented unit because its efficiency had lapsed in the interim. Ironing out these and other difficulties at his hospital caused him a great deal of concern and anxiety, and I am sure that these stresses also contributed to his coronary.

Furthermore, because of all this, he had no time for regular exercise. For years he had played a good, hard game of tennis most Sunday mornings, but because of the preparations for the trip and the build-up of work and tension on our return, the routine had been disrupted. He did sail at the weekends, but to race on Saturdays he had to rush all morning in order to get home and be on the boat in time for the start.

He was also very much overweight. He is a man who enjoys good food and I enjoy cooking. Although a small-breakfast eater, at hospital during the day there are cups of tea plus cakes or sandwiches continually, and at night he always had a big meal. He adored butter on vegetables and lashings of cream on desserts. When he was taken ill he must have weighed nearly fifteen kilograms more than he should have.

I wondered that night, as so many partners in similar circumstances must do, whether I would ever have him beside me again, and asked the question that must be typical: Why has this thing happened to us?

It helps a little to know that coronaries attack people in all walks of life—unskilled workers, white-collar workers, business and professional people, farmers, executives. No-one seems to have found any one definite cause, but cardiologists working in different parts of the world have established a number of "contributing causes". Family history is one: if a person's parents have suffered from heart disease it would appear that he or she is more likely to be affected than another whose parents have not. Overeating, eating the wrong foods, cigarette smoking, insufficient exercise—all these, and of course any combination of them, are culprits, and when aggravated by great stress, there is a high probability that the condition will occur.

—Norma held a highly charged executive position, involving dealings with the public, night-time meetings following a day's work and not always popular decision-making. She had a devoted husband

and children and a pleasant social life. She was overweight and had high blood pressure, a condition from which both her parents had suffered. A period of great stress and tension, added to these, precipitated her coronary.

—Jim had a sheep station out west. Thin and spare, leading the fairly leisurely life of the country man, a smoker but not to excess, he was the last person one would expect to have a coronary. But both his parents and several other members of his family had suffered from heart disease.

—Harold was a businessman. He played bowls, but that was almost his only exercise. He enjoyed rich food, but did not keep late hours and had plenty of rest. He suffered a mild coronary.

—Don was not yet forty when he was stricken. A busy general practitioner, interested in life and fond of tennis, he was a little overweight, he smoked about thirty cigarettes a day, and sometimes worked fourteen to fifteen hours a day. He rushed through his house calls to be in time for surgery hours, tried to read up his medical journals, attend clinical meetings at hospitals, and still make time for his family. When he was taken to hospital his wife, normally a very sensible and practical young woman, almost went to pieces. For her it was almost the last straw when a well-meaning acquaintance, intending to ask after her husband's health, said, "Whatever have you been doing to Don?"

This is something that all partners of those who have suffered coronaries have to face: Have I done this to my partner? Is it my fault? And it is a question to which most people answer no. No, I begged him or her not to work so hard, not to play so hard, not to smoke so much, to lose some weight.

It is not a coincidence that there is practically no heart disease, and certainly not these sudden coronary occlusions, among primitive peoples. They do not overeat, nor do they eat a lot of sophisticated foods. They have sufficient exercise—they don't drive everywhere, they walk; they swim, fish, hunt, climb trees. They are not always in a hurry to get things done or to get to places; if not today—well, tomorrow, or next week. There are not people always "at" them wanting them to sit on this committee, or see this patient or client or customer, or placate this dissatisfied person. If they smoke, it is not to excess, because tobacco is expensive or not readily available.

Coronaries occur in the affluent society, and in Australia more people between forty and sixty-five die from this than from any other cause. However, once a person has had a coronary, the partner, realising what has contributed to it, can help them rearrange their life to minimise excess stress, both mental and physical, and eliminate overeating and smoking so that they may go on to live to a ripe old age.

Meanwhile, the patient is immobilised in hospital.

CHAPTER 3

And Then—

The next day I went to the hospital, armed with the necessary extra pyjamas, a transistor radio, toilet gear, and books. He looked much better, but very tired.

"Once that pain went, I was right," he said, but he knew he would have to stay in hospital for some time.

Beside his bed was the paraphernalia of an intensive care unit—oxygen cylinder, electronic monitoring equipment, etcetera—a rather terrifying and subduing array, but reassuring, when I thought about it, how they were geared for any emergency.

Meanwhile there were arrangements to cancel and others to make. Because we were officially on holiday he had no professional commitments for the immediate future. The next time I visited I was to bring his diary and he would tell me what to do about operations and consultations booked for the next few weeks. His doctor said that all his honorary work at hospitals would have to be discontinued for at least three months, and he would not make any decisions at this stage about private work.

Now, a specialist usually works alone, and other doctors refer patients to him. If a doctor in a group practice is taken ill his partners are still working and he still receives a share of the earnings, but if a man working solo suddenly stops, so does his income. This was something neither of us had considered. Bills would still have to be paid. My husband had a sickness and accident insurance policy, so the company was duly notified. This payment would help—when it was made. Such things take some time. Of course there would be money coming in from patients seen earlier in the year—though gradually, because people tend to leave doctors' bills until after the Christmas holidays. However, we were not going to worry unduly over this; he just had to rest and recover completely.

We had made a few holiday arrangements with friends. We had planned to spend New Year's Eve moored in a bay with friends who also had their boat in Pittwater, we had arranged to take another couple out for the day on New Year's Day, one day we were to come ashore at Newport for a luncheon with some other friends at their beach house, and so on. All these people had to be phoned and told what had happened. Various members of the family and close friends had to know also. Ringing people up to tell them, going through the tale over and over again, I found extremely exhausting. And of course this was followed up, day after day, by their kindly phoning to inquire. People who had just heard the news phoned to express their concern—and wanted to hear all the details.

Then there was the great problem of what to do about our daughter, who was in Italy studying and enjoying herself hugely. Devoted to her daddy, she would come home immediately if I cabled her. But as he was apparently out of danger, would this be fair to her? Also, if she came galloping home, mightn't he think he was much worse than he actually was? I discussed this with his doctor. He agreed with me that it was unnecessary to bring her home unless my husband was fretting for her and really wanted her back. Fortunately he brought up the subject himself.

"I don't want her to come home before she's ready, just because of me," he said. "I'll write to her in a few days and tell her I'm in hospital, but she's not to worry."

He wrote, but it happened that there was quite a lot of industrial unrest in Italy at that time. It was three weeks before we heard from her. Later she told us that she had written as soon as she had received the letter, but in the meantime he asked every day whether there was a letter from her and every day I had to say no. He became rather upset at her apparent lack of sympathy, and I became upset because he was upset. It was a fortnight before I was able to put pen to paper to tell her exactly what had happened and when I had finished I felt completely wrung out. Of course, when her letters began arriving they were full of cheer-ups and jokes, and several came within the space of a few days.

At first our son and I were the only visitors allowed, but eventually relatives and friends could come. Many of his colleagues would drop in for a few minutes, especially those attending Royal Prince Alfred Hospital. People were most kind, sending books, flowers, fruit and "get well" cards. He was in hospital over New Year, and all those patients well enough were allowed to have a little drink to celebrate. I think he had a better New Year's Eve than I did!

Once the holiday weekend was over, it was necessary for me to arrange alternatives for the work previously booked. His colleagues were really

18

wonderful. One undertook to see and operate on any patients that could not wait until he returned to work. The authorities at his own hospital began discussing ways to lighten his work-load, appointing a staff surgeon to take over some of the public work that he had been doing in an honorary capacity and which he felt he would have to relinquish when he returned. As his condition began to improve, those involved would call to see him and talk over these policies.

At this stage of his recovery he began to ask for journals and case reports to be brought to him. Several times a week his secretary and I would go through his mail and I would take to him for instructions any matters that we could not deal with. This was approved as good occupational therapy. Just the same, time in hospital lagged for him. We hired a television set, which he enjoyed for the sporting coverage, the news and certain other selected programmes. I took him his painting gear and occasionally he would spend some hours, completely relaxed, with a picture. I took in the Scrabble set and most evenings after the news we would have a game together.

All this time he was on the strictest of diets to reduce his weight and consequently the load on his heart. I was instructed as to the foods he might and might not eat. Cream, butter—animal fats of all kinds—were completely forbidden. His meat intake was limited, and such cuts as lamb chops with a lot of fat had to be avoided. I was given booklets of advice and recipes suitable for his diet. Every few days biochemical tests were taken, which included examinations of the blood cholesterol level. This was another reason for the fat-free diet, and also for the very limited number of eggs allowed—two per week.

Fortunately he had always been a light smoker, enjoying only four or five cigarettes a day, mostly after a meal or in the evening if relaxing at home, so the edict to stop completely made little difference to him.

After about a week he was allowed out of bed, to go to the bathroom, to sit in a chair, and to walk a little in the hospital corridor. This was the stage when he began to be concerned with the future. Would he be able to operate again? What kind of life would he have? And this was the stage when our dear friend John came, one afternoon while I was there, and sat down, saying quietly and seriously, "Now I want to tell you a few things."

I was apprehensive. What would we hear? The risks of future attacks? A bad outlook? My own heart sank into my shoes. However, he began, "About twenty years ago, old Charles had a coronary like yours."

We knew "old Charles" led a busy professional life and had an interesting social life, travelled quite often, and held office in professional organisations. This piece of information cheered us both considerably.

John spoke of several other people, mostly doctors whom we both knew as busy men leading full and satisfying lives, all of whom had at some time during the previous fifteen years suffered a coronary. This information had a quite inspiring effect upon us; the future was not so bleak after all. In fact, provided my husband could reduce his work-load and his weight, it now appeared quite good. The quarter-hour visit from this wonderful, quiet physician was one of the best morale-boosters of my experience.

At least two friends who have had similar coronaries during the last year—and their spouses—have had to face the same problem as ours: with a daughter overseas, what is the best to do? In each case they tackled it the same way as we did. Actually it would probably be better, if possible, to send a reassuring cable asking the girl to phone home; this would eliminate any worries caused by mail delays. Our own daughter returned home eighteen months later and began to do her share of "watching over Dad". One of the other girls also returned and after staying at home in the country for a while came to the city, with her father's blessing, to work and enjoy a fuller and more interesting life. There is no doubt that their homecoming brought some of the light back to their fathers' eyes.

All sorts of financial matters can be a worry to someone in hospital too. Most self-employed people have a sickness and accident insurance policy, as my husband did; most people who are employed would be covered by sick leave; and all hospitals have trained social workers to help patients and their families solve any problems of this nature. But there are other problems connected with money.

Mr Johnson had his coronary towards the end of June, and his worries about his income-tax return were interfering with his progress until his son mentioned the matter to his doctor. Of course it needed only an application to the Deputy Commissioner for an extension to be granted until he was able to cope with the return.

Mr Roberts was worried about some business matters that really needed his personal attention. His doctor considered it the lesser of two evils to let his mind work on the business in question, rather than have him worrying because it was incomplete. Once he had made his decisions and delegated the remainder of the work he was able to relax and rest properly.

Mr Jackson was worried about his hire-purchase commitments on his car, furniture, and electrical equipment. The hospital social worker advised his wife to contact the hire-purchase companies concerned and a satisfactory solution was worked out.

Sometimes, too, there is trouble with landlords over late rent payments. If people are living in a Housing Commission home the rent is automatically adjusted by the government, but if they rent privately and have difficulties the hospital social worker once again can help in overcoming them.

In all cases where extra stress is considered a triggering factor in the coronary, naturally the question of reducing the work-load is raised. And efforts are made to help the patient cope with worries when they finally have to be faced again.

Some patients will talk over these worries with their partners while still in hospital, but some will bottle it all up, realising the partner is concerned enough already with the illness, the constant trips to hospital, coping with phone calls and visitors, and with the family generally. As well, they feel frustration at not being allowed to do things for themselves and having to depend so much on others. These people become very irritable so that, of course, the partner is *not* helped. Strained already, they may not understand the patient's impatience with them or sudden flashes of anger towards them, and consequently they worry all the more. It would really be better for them both if the patient discussed things with the partner.

Many partners feel that the doctor is there to treat the patient physically and do not realise that psychological treatment is also important. If the doctor does not know about matters that are worrying the patient or the partner he or she obviously cannot help—either with advice, reassurance, or by referring them to someone else such as the social worker. It is important, therefore, for the partner to discuss these problems and not take the attitude of their being too small a matter to worry the doctor with.

There is also no doubt that when a person is in hospital, wondering what the future holds, it is a tremendous help in settling anxieties and expediting recovery to hear of others who have experienced the same illness and doubts as to their capabilities afterwards and who are now leading normal, active lives. As soon as patients realise that once the immediate need for rest and treatment is past they can progressively return to a normal life, their own mental state improves remarkably and their families can heave a sigh of relief. They will not be invalids or semi-invalids indefinitely!

CHAPTER 4

Home Again

After nearly three weeks in hospital the doctor one day said, "Well, you can go home in a few days."

In our house the bedrooms are all upstairs, but there is a utility room off the kitchen and we can put a bed in there if necessary. I mentioned this, expressing my concern about the stairs, but I was told that it would not hurt him at all to go upstairs, that he had been walking around the corridors of the hospital quite a lot, and that provided he went slowly and not too many times a day, it would actually be good for him. He would be happier in his own bed, too.

It would be necessary for him to take a mild sedative at night and anti-coagulant tablets to minimise the chance of any recurrence. He was also to do some exercises, described in a booklet provided by the National Heart Foundation and somewhat similar to the Canadian Air Force 5BX. These were started a few at a time and gradually increased until he was spending ten to fifteen minutes each day doing some apparently quite strenuous ones. I couldn't do those press-ups—and I was healthy! He had also to walk, beginning with short distances that gradually increased to about two kilometres a day. Mostly we would walk together in the late afternoon or early evening, and it really was very pleasant.

There was also, of course, the strict diet. It became a challenge to me to make interesting, tasty meals within the restrictions. The *Anti-Coronary Cookbook* and some recipes provided by Royal Prince Alfred Hospital were a help, but mostly I used my ingenuity—I think this was good occupational therapy for me! Meat was limited to small amounts of lean beef or veal; liver, kidney and brains were permitted only occasionally; shellfish were allowed only once a week. Chicken and fish, however, could be eaten as often as he liked.

I found all sorts of interesting, inexpensive canned fish—herrings in wine, in beer, in lemon sauce, and gefüllte fish from Israel—that along with sardines, salmon and pilchards could be added to salads for lunches. Fresh fish I either grilled (using polyunsaturated margarine, as recommended by the hospital, instead of butter) or steamed—adding parsley—or baked with tomatoes. Chicken could be steamed, grilled, or prepared as a casserole with wine or mushrooms and onions.

The only salad restrictions were that mayonnaise, unless made with polyunsaturated oil, and such fattening things as potato salad were to be avoided. The only cheese permitted was cottage cheese, and this we sometimes incorporated in salads with prunes, celery, gherkins, pears or pineapple.

We experimented with different types of low-calorie biscuits—Vita-Weat, Ryvita, Norwegian flat-bread, etcetera—as a substitute for bread and found them quite adequate.

My husband missed potatoes with dinner, but he soon adapted to carrots, parsnips, pumpkin or choko instead. About once a week I would allow a potato with a baked dinner. One of my problems was that we all adore baked dinners and it seemed, with the diet restrictions, that they might not be allowed. I talked to the dietitian before my husband left hospital and learned that if potatoes, pumpkin, and other vegetables are fried in polyunsaturated oil instead of being baked in dripping around the meat, in the old-fashioned way, they look the same, are crisp, and there is very little difference in the flavour. I baked the meat in the Continental way, standing it on a grid over a dish containing water. The meat was seasoned with salt and pepper and the appropriate herbs or garlic. I bought corner pieces of topside beef because it is less fatty than rolled rib or sirloin, and I usually marinated it in a little red wine, basted it with wine, and cooked it very slowly. The family was really enthusiastic about this.

For desserts, cream and ice-cream were out. Often we had fresh fruit but sometimes it was nice to have a proper "pud". As eggwhites were not limited I sometimes made meringues or flummeries. Jellies, too, were appreciated.

Breakfasts were usually fruit followed by fish, cottage cheese, the occasional egg, tomatoes, mushrooms or eggplant, plus a slice of toast with marmalade or honey.

We had to be very strict about between-meal snacks. There were to be no cakes or biscuits, except perhaps, as a special treat, biscuits made with polyunsaturated margarine, and then only if there were not going to be potatoes that night, or if he had had only one slice of bread all day. As he was allowed alcohol in moderation we continued our custom of a pre-dinner drink, but the titbits with it were very much limited.

When my husband first came home from hospital he would stay in bed until after breakfast then get up and do his exercises, have a leisurely shower, and dress. (Getting into clothes instead of pyjamas is a great morale-builder.) By this time it would be mid-morning and he would come downstairs. Depending on the weather, he would sit outside or indoors, or perhaps water the garden. We are fortunate in that our front verandah gets the morning sun and the nor'-easters and is shaded in the afternoon, while the back verandah gets the afternoon sun, the southerly and westerly winds, and is cool in the mornings. At the side of the house there is a flagged terrace. So I would vary where we ate lunch, setting a table where it was most suitable. I bought two cheap, lightweight duralumin chairs to save moving the heavier outdoor furniture around; these he could carry himself without effort, which made him feel more independent. This changing of the scene was, I think, quite helpful in combating boredom.

After lunch there was always a rest, either downstairs or in the bedroom. Quite often he would have visitors, and there was television, records to play, books, magazines, and papers to read. If no friends called we would usually have a game of Scrabble during the afternoon, when he had returned to bed.

The length of time he was up each day increased progressively— from three to four hours at first until after about ten days he was staying up for dinner and going to bed after the 7 p.m. news. He did a few little jobs around the house that involved no great effort such as mending things with glue (I'm hopeless at that sort of thing), unpacking the dishwasher, cutting up meat for the dog and the cat, and painting the doors of the kitchen cupboards — all with much encouragement!

After about a week he was allowed out in the car, if someone else was driving. It was summertime and some days were very hot. I asked if I could take him to the beach occasionally and his doctor said yes, provided he did not get buffeted by the surf, or go for any long swims. He could certainly have a dip and cool off in the water, or relax on the beach. This made a very welcome change. On Saturday afternoons we would drive to Bradley's Head or Cremorne Point to watch the sailing races and after being home for about a fortnight he was allowed to go to a film once a week — the late-afternoon session. We chose a few really good escapist films. Sometimes our son and a friend would accompany us.

This was all a great advance from the first few days and nights he was home. At that time I scarcely slept. I was frightened to move in bed in case I disturbed him. I would surreptitiously watch his breathing and gently feel his pulse. If he was at all restless I was filled with alarm.

At last he was told he could drive his car himself but only locally at first and if someone was with him.

To many patients, being able to drive again is a milestone in their recovery. When Colin, an engineer, was stricken by his coronary he resented being driven. He had refused to allow his seventeen-year-old son to drive until he had finished school, but now his wife sent the lad to the local driving school for lessons so that in an emergency there would be another driver in the family. It also meant that someone else could go shopping for food. Of course Colin himself now drives and leads a normal life.

To others who are accustomed to mowing the lawn themselves, the fact that this is forbidden for a time seems almost like an attack on their competence. They hate to see a partner cutting the grass, or if their children take on the task, they worry about accidents occurring. I understand that if a person is recovering satisfactorily from a mild coronary and has been a keen gardener, the doctor will sometimes prescribe exercises that resemble pushing a lawnmower so that after a few weeks at home, if he wishes to cut the grass himself he can, and his family, knowing that his muscles and heart have been prepared for this by the exercises, do not have to worry that he is overstraining himself. Hard mowing with a hand mower — uphill, or in very rough grass — would probably not be allowed at first. Under these circumstances a motor mower is a good invest-ment.

The question of sexual intercourse worries many couples. Mostly they are diffident about raising it with their doctors. Partners may hold themselves aloof, thinking that the excitement would be bad for the patient and that all sorts of problems could then arise. They have been emotionally upset by the whole situation — the suddenness of the illness, the alteration in their way of life, the worry about a recurrence — and now would like to be complete partners again but fear the consequences. Often patients do not understand all this; they know they have recovered greatly when they are sent home, although they also know they must be careful about many things. And they, too, are often worried about the future and a bit "browned-off" with being confined. They are apt to mistake their partners' motives, thinking, perhaps, that they are not loved as before because they are invalided at the moment; they may wonder about their sexuality, or think that their partners are doubting them. So, added to the problems of adjustment is that of sexual frustration.

Some coronaries are much more serious than others; consequently the return to normal activities of all forms varies from patient to patient. It is therefore important for both man and woman, and their future relationship, that they ask the doctor when every aspect of their life together can return to normal and also how gradual this should be. After all, your own happiness is controlled by the amount of tension between you.

Boredom at home can be overcome in a number of ways. Apart from the obvious diversions of reading, radio, television and visitors, you can encourage interest in a new hobby. Perhaps the patient has always been interested in art and might like to try drawing or painting. There are teach-yourself books to be bought at reasonable prices. For the non-creative in this field there are painting-by-numbers sets which become quite absorbing and are attractive when completed.

The patient might like to take up the guitar, mandolin or piano. None of these is strenuous and all are interesting. Once again there are teach-yourself books, or it might be possible to arrange for a teacher to give a few lessons. The patient might have always wanted to be a writer but has never had time to attempt it. If he or she has difficulty in putting down thoughts on paper, there are a number of very interesting correspondence courses available. These courses can be most rewarding, and the assignments fill in an hour or two each day. There is always the chance that in the end a new feature-writer, short-story-writer or novelist will have emerged!

Handicrafts such as weaving, knitting, leather-work or basket-making all help to pass the time creatively. The occupational therapist at the hospital can often give good advice about these activities. And most homes have odd jobs waiting to be done that do not require a lot of energy: a skirting-board to be painted, power plugs to be changed, knives to be sharpened, things to be mended.

My husband and I enjoy an occasional game of cards. One of our friends suggested he might like a game of bridge. Her husband was able to leave his business early, so several times they came to see us at about 5 p.m. and we would play for a couple of hours, then I would serve something to eat. My husband could still go to bed early after having had a pleasant, returning-to-normal session. Another person may be keen on crossword puzzles, while another may like jigsaw puzzles. But if your partner likes doing things with other people, he or she might learn bridge or solo.

Generally speaking, as much of one's normal life as possible interspersed with a little variety each day, plus frequent rests, seems to be a good recipe for a normal convalescence.

CHAPTER 5

Now, the Problems

I realise we were fortunate, in that my husband's coronary was a mild one, that we did not have very pressing financial problems, that he had many interests to counteract the boredom of enforced inactivity, and that he knew he would eventually be able to return to his work with the load reduced and with the cooperation of his colleagues. As a doctor he knew that provided he was careful in the future he need never have another attack, and although this was one worry that I had, he eventually reassured me.

Despite all this there were many times when my husband would appear depressed and become irritated by something we would consider a minor matter. I can remember occasions when a battle seemed imminent over things like our son's haircut, or the clothes he was wearing, and my son would come to me, quite upset, saying, "Gee, Mum, what's biting Dad? He's just so unreasonable; he gets so upset about a little thing like that." I would point out that if it was such a little thing perhaps he could do his hair, or put on shoes, or remedy whatever was the cause of the trouble so that Dad would not get annoyed.

Sometimes my husband would take things I said the wrong way. Many times I fought back tears and the desire to reply sharply. Often, later, he would apologise for his ill humour, admitting that the matter had not been very important and that he should not allow himself to get so annoyed so easily. I think he realised that he was being unfair to us, but of course a patient's family, being the closest to him and with him more than other people, are naturally the ones to be snarled at first.

As he became stronger we would sometimes discuss this, especially after a flare-up. Usually it would have occurred because something was worrying him—perhaps his future activities, how soon he could return to work, how much he would be able to do. He had lost some of his self-confidence and he also became tired very quickly. The daily rest was not merely to fill in time; it was really necessary.

Since he has been back at work we have found the same thing: he seems to become tired more easily, and if he does not stop to rest he becomes irritable. I learnt to assess the situation and even now will often tell him that there's time for him to rest and read the paper before dinner, and purposely keep the meal late to give him a chance to settle down. At other times I will ask if something is bothering him, and often in talking over some problem with me he finds the tension goes. Sometimes we solve the problem by discussing it; sometimes, if it is the management of a sick patient that is worrying him, just to tell me about it is enough.

However, it is impossible to remove all tension and annoyance from one's life; there are external irritations such as late mail and non-delivery of newspapers, and tensions caused by lack of consideration by others, especially the younger members of the family. One big crisis arose when our son, who like many other boys his age is mad about old cars, bought a 1942 ex-army jeep, with his father's consent. It was cheap and unregistered, and he and his friends spent months reconditioning it with the idea of using it as a "beach buggy" and, I suppose, eventually selling it at an enormous profit. One of his friends had a welding kit and undertook to cut the rusty parts from the body and replace them with new metal. Unfortunately he was not the most reliable person and while waiting for this part of the job to be finished, my son suddenly appeared one Saturday morning with a similar-vintage Harley-Davidson motorcycle and sidecar. As he has a good job and can save quite a lot of his salary, such transactions do not involve us at all, so I didn't know the thing had arrived until my husband stormed into the house, absolutely livid. His "Do you know what's on the front lawn?" was the first I knew of it.

Well, he really went to town about this. At last I begged him to calm down. He decreed that the bike had to be off the premises by the end of the weekend — or else! (We didn't ask, "Or else, what?") Very chastened, our son began phoning any friends who had large garages or spare space, trying to find somewhere to store the thing. Finally someone agreed to stow it under their back verandah provided his mother did not object. I heard our son say, "I thought my Dad was going to have another heart attack, he was so mad."

Later I tackled my husband, insisting that he should not get so cross. Grinning, he admitted that he was not nearly as annoyed as he had sounded, but he thought it unreasonable to have another vehicle in a thousand pieces around the place while the first one was unfinished and he really wanted to get the message over. Well, I suppose he was entitled to express his annoyance, but I am not sure that he should have traded on the family's fears of another attack. On the other hand, it was pure thoughtlessness on our son's part not to have discussed the new project with his father first just as he had discussed the jeep.

Most partners notice that coronary patients become irritable much more easily after their attack. It requires quite a lot of self-restraint, when you are feeling overwrought, not to retaliate sharply, and it is difficult not to feel hurt when one is picked on, or defensive when the children are picked on.

We took another keen sailor and his wife out on our boat recently. It was his first sail since his coronary and although they were both obviously enjoying themselves, he seemed to be picking on her all the time. "Don't be so silly, Mary; *that's* the jib sheet." "For goodness' sake, Mary, pull on that rope." "Whatever are you doing that for, Mary?" And so on. She took it all, with murmured apologies for being stupid. I hope, as he progresses, that she will begin to answer back, because it is not good for anybody to be a martyr to a partner's irritability.

Sometimes young children become extremely naughty when their father is around all the time. Perhaps they resent their mother's divided attention. Perhaps they feel insecure; they may have overheard their parents discussing money worries or the possibility of another attack. Sometimes these children develop acute behaviour problems as a result; it is important that parents inform their children's teachers of the troubles at home. Teenagers may react very strongly to the change in their parents' demeanour, even leaving home because they cannot cope with these additional problems.

Usually the patient's doctor warns both patient and partner about the side-effects of depression and anxiety so the family will be prepared and not take the irritability too seriously. They realise that the patient is upset at his or her dependence on others and does not mean to be so bad-tempered. However, some people take this dependence very badly indeed.

Mrs Allen went out to work temporarily to help pay the family bills. She was lucky that, after discussing it with her husband, he understood that she was not belittling him and was merely removing some of the strain.

Mrs Barnes was not so fortunate. She took a part-time job while the children were at school, and would leave a prepared lunch for her husband. However, he was bitterly resentful. He resented being left alone for all those hours and then having to share her attention with the children, who naturally expected Mum to listen to their school gossip and give them afternoon tea as usual. He resented being asked to prepare the vegetables and, later, to do some household shopping and chores that he considered women's work, while his wife was usurping his position as the breadwinner.

When Bill, a farmer, returned home his grown-up son was managing the property very efficiently and using some rather more modern ideas than Bill himself would have employed. While acknowledging the good job being done, Bill was full of worries about the financial commitment involved in the improvements even though both the son and his accountant explained

36

that the worries were groundless. The transfer of control tended to make Bill very irritable with his family.

While it is natural for a patient to be anxious about the future and depressed about the present inactivity, it does not seem altogether fair that the family should suffer because of increased irritability. It would seem that some patients are irritable because they feel insecure and do not know what is happening but there are others who do know, and resent it, and in this case the irritability is a form of "getting back" at the world which the patient considers has done him or her a bad turn. Don't be a martyr! React as you would normally. If you do not they will either become tyrants or think they are much worse than they really are. By the time they are home from hospital it is no longer necessary to avoid *all* tension, and it is far better to discuss together things that worry *you*, as well as things that worry *him* or *her*, than to let additional and unnecessary tension build up.

If patients are not progressing as rapidly as they should, doctors will frequently refer them to the National Heart Foundation's rehabilitation units. Patients, and their families, are given advice and aid to help them cope with the problems of lack of self-confidence and anxiety over the future. Do not hesitate to discuss your partner's progress with the doctor.

Underlying the problems in most cases is the fact that the patient is at home all the time and needing the partner. However, many couples find that the period of convalescence at home brings them closer to each other than they have been for years. It is a period of readjustment for them both, and it can be a period of becoming reacquainted with each other, of reassessment, and perhaps of changes in their personal relationship.

Unless the man works at home or is at some stage of retirement, the pattern of the lives of most couples is that the man goes off to work in the mornings and is occupied all day and sometimes in the evening with activities in which the woman usually has very little part, while she is involved with the home, the family, perhaps a job, and whatever other interests fill her day. Most evenings are spent together, but in many homes a large part of the time is given to watching television or reading, and there is not much conversation; or they may go out to see other people or to some form of entertainment. Some weekends might be spent doing things together but often the man spends at least half a day either participating in, or watching, sport. Suddenly, when he or she returns from hospital, they find they must spend more time in each other's company than perhaps at any other time in their lives. And this has varied effects on them both.

Many couples have said how much they have enjoyed this enforced "togetherness" — how it felt like a perpetual holiday, how for the first time they really have had the pleasure of each other's company through not having to rush away to something, and how much fun they have had together as the patient has been able to do progressively more. But other couples have found, to their dismay, that they have talked on a mundane level for so many years that now they do not know what to say to each other; they hardly know each other. Some of these people rise to the occasion, and buy them was difficult, with Alan and the children all needing her attention. So if friends offer to bring a cake or some biscuits with them, do not be too proud to accept. They will feel that they are helping and you will not feel so hassled.

This is the time, too, when true kindness and friendship manifest themselves, when people one has considered merely as friendly acquaintances sometimes show themselves to be capable of greater sympathy and assistance than others with whom one was on more intimate terms and considered close, either as family or friends. One does not forget the helpfulness of others in one's time of need: some people have told me of their disappointment with the reactions — or lack of same — of friends and relatives.

Certainly visits, phone calls, letters and "get well" cards all help the convalescent patient accustomed to activity to become reconciled to a period of restriction. That period varies from patient to patient, depending on whether there were any complicating factors during or after the operation, the person's general physical condition, age, etcetera, and also on the patient's mental attitude to returning to normal life.

It is important for families to encourage the patient to do as much as he or she feels able to do (if permitted — for example, no driving for a certain period), while ensuring that these activities are not a strain on chest, legs or back. This applies also to sexual activity. The general advice usually given is that once the patient feels like it, then sexual relations may resume — this is usually after about three or four weeks at home. The convalescent should understand, however, that the partner may still be physically and/or mentally wrung out from the emotional strain of coping. The extra tasks at home and the many phone calls and visitors are also wearying.

Some people find the white stockings, designed to protect and support their legs, irritating and refuse to wear them. These people must therefore take more care not to knock the scars and hurt their legs. They are likely to have more trouble with swollen ankles. A feeling of numbness or "pins and needles" affects people sometimes: rubbing the legs often helps disperse this.

One problem some people face when the convalescent patient comes home from hospital is the "no smoking" edict. Cigarette smoking is labelled Public Enemy No. 1 as regards health hazards, with risks of lung cancer as well as heart disease. In hospital neither patients nor visitors are permitted to smoke, but once the patient goes home the craving for a cigarette by a habitual smoker is sometimes overwhelming. If the partner is a smoker then it is doubly difficult, not only for the convalescent but also for the partner—he or she may want to help the patient, but cannot and feels very guilty about it. There are several self-help schemes for addicted smokers—programmes such as "Quit for Life"—and information about these is available from the State Health Department, the Cancer Council, or the National Heart Foundation.

During this convalescent period at home many people reassess their lifestyles. They work out priorities and the relative importance of some of their accustomed activities.

Bruce, whose bypass operation took place when he was in his early forties, was a highly motivated, ambitious man who used to work long hours and go home late for dinner. He decided he was not seeing enough of his young children, then in primary school—his wife used to give them their evening meal early and often they were already in bed when their father came home. He decided that once he was back at work he would come home earlier so that they could have family dinners together. However, he was impatient with the rate of his recovery and at times was extremely irritable. As Bruce had never suffered a coronary, but had gone to surgery following an attack of chest pain and abnormal results from an exercise ECG and angiogram, he was worried about his future. Until he became stronger and realised that he could continue with his life's work, there was a strained relationship between him and his wife. She felt he resented her monitoring his meals, his rest periods, his visitors: later they were able to communicate more easily.

Often, as with patients recovering from coronaries, a period of convalescence at home is a chance for partners to resume a companionship which during the years has diminished for various reasons: it can be a time of great revival of affection and understanding.

If you do have any worries relating to a convalescent patient's rehabilitation, do not hesitate to consult the rehabilitation officer at the hospital in which he or she was a patient. Also, National Heart Foundation offices in Sydney and Melbourne have trained people available to give advice on a wide range of concerns —from employment and social security, to travelling, and coping with personal depression or changed relationships. Anyone can phone for advice and assistance in an informal way: it is not necessary to go through the procedure of making appointments.

For medical problems, of course, consult your doctor.

CHAPTER 14

Some Landmarks in Recovery

My husband needed his afternoon rest for several weeks. Every day he began doing more, walking further—gradually returning to normal life.

The first sign occurred after he had been home about two weeks when he said, "Tonight I am going to take you out to dinner."

We went to a local restaurant and that outing was really a landmark in his recovery. I was a little doubtful about going out so soon after the operation, but he felt confident and it certainly was pleasant for me to have a holiday from planning and preparing meals. Organising three meals a day at home when one is accustomed to a busy life is a challenge, but it is also a tie and time-consuming.

After that outing we began visiting friends for small intimate dinners, making sure that he had a good rest during the day and that we did not stay out too late. Sometimes one or two friends would come and have a meal with us. Seeing people like this, in a more normal fashion instead of as a convalescent, was very good for his morale.

On our return from overseas a number of invitations had been waiting. Decisions had to be made about these. Some it was not possible to accept. One invitation was for an afternoon wedding to be held about six weeks after his operation. The bride's mother told me it would not be a large affair and that the "breakfast" would be a sit-down high tea. My husband's cardiologist gave him permission to attend. At the wedding there were several people who had already undergone bypass surgery and were obviously very well. This was most encouraging to my husband, especially when Joan told him she entered and completed the course for the City to Surf Competition— walking, not running—only nine months after her bypass operation!

That wedding marked the beginning of his return to social life. The following week friends had arranged a party to celebrate a fiftieth birthday. We went, enjoyed it, and the crowd of people there did not worry my husband. Actually, he received much attention from those who either had not known about his operation or had not had a chance to visit him.

After that party we accepted invitations provided that we were not going out too many nights in a week and that the outings would not be too hectic.

We began making general outings more interesting. At the Art Gallery we caught the final days of an exhibition of Elioth Gruner's paintings and later in his convalescence there was a marvellous exhibition of Aboriginal bark paintings. Walking around the gallery and looking at art works was a change from just walking for exercise—and it was still walking. Sometimes we would drive to the Botanic Gardens or to one of the beaches and we would walk in different surroundings.

I booked seats for a theatre matinee during the third week he was home from hospital. He found sitting in a theatre seat no problem, so we were able to go to plays again. We had booked months before for Dame Janet Baker's concerts and when the time came, about four weeks after he came home, I asked him if he would like me to arrange for him to use the lift at the Opera House, a suggestion met with derision! Of course he could manage the Opera House steps! And he did — easily. Afterwards, walking to the car which was parked halfway up a hill, he took great pride in the fact that not once did he need to stop and rest on the way. This was in great contrast to his physical condition for the year or so before his bypass when we would walk slowly, with pauses from time to time. I knew he needed these stops and sometimes I would pretend that I was tired or say my high-heeled shoes were troubling me if I saw him looking weary and strained.

"I would not have done that six months ago!" became a frequent exclamation during these next few weeks.

Before we left for overseas we had made plans to join a National Trust country weekend. This was scheduled to occur seven weeks after his operation, and before final arrangements were made for such a long drive he needed clearance from his cardiologist. This was readily given. By that time his surgeon had checked him over and was pleased that everything was going so well and my husband had driven himself to an early morning appointment with his cardiologist, using a small towel as a protective pad between the seat belt and his chest.

Normally on long drives we share the driving. For this country weekend I had intended to do it all, but he said he felt he could do some of the driving and he did, with no ill effects. That weekend was a great success, another landmark in his recovery. He managed, without any trouble, visits to interesting properties specially open for the National Trust, wine-tastings at nearby vineyards, even the somewhat chaotic catering at arranged lunches. Each afternoon we returned to the motel and he rested. On the Saturday night there was a dinner-dance. For years, if we went to such a function (and it was rare), once the dinner was finished and the band began to play he would say, "Come on, let's go." But this evening when the band began to play he said, "Come on, let's dance!" I was amazed and delighted. I love dancing and had forgone this activity for so long. As we danced he said, "I bet you didn't think we'd be doing this." That was another landmark in his recovery.

After the first month at home he had left off his white stockings at night and by the time we went to the country he had discarded them completely.

He continued to wake in the night and needed to take digesics for several weeks. He was also taking one aspirin tablet each day as a precaution against blood clotting, which could cause problems.

Once he could drive again he began going to the hospital for meetings, to check mail, or to see a few patients. He was delighted to be back to his professional activities, especially seeing patients again. He told me that at one stage, a few months earlier, he had wondered whether he ever would. Each week he was able to do a little more, although it was about ten weeks before he began working normal hours and performing operations.

Another landmark was the first dinner party at

home since the operation. There were eight people, a comfortable number to seat around our dining table. Acting the host did not worry him at all. It was a happy evening and after our guests had departed I suggested, as had been my custom for several years, that he should go to bed and leave me to clear up at my leisure. I prefer to do this. My dinner parties are always easy-catering and easy-serving kinds but there is always an accumulation of plates, cutlery and glasses in the kitchen and really only one person can pack a dish-washer. Usually I leave any pots or casserole dishes to soak until the next day. On this occasion he said, "No. You've been doing so much. I'm going to stay up and help you." So he put chairs back in place, brought out the coffee cups, and did jobs like that while I cleared the kitchen, then he insisted on drying up the things that required hand-washing. It was great—just like years ago. Instead of his being asleep by the time I went upstairs, we were able to chat about the evening together.

It took quite a long time for me to stop watching over him as earnestly as during the previous few years. I was so accustomed to observing him, whispering, "Are you all right?" from time to time, that I found I was still doing this. It amused him. Finally I stopped, as he would always respond, "Yes, I'm quite all right. Don't forget I've got new coronary arteries now."

Another landmark was resuming tennis. Once or twice during his convalescence he came with me, watched us playing, chatted with those waiting to play, and had coffee with us—a kind of social outing. On the Sunday after our return from the National Trust weekend, about eight weeks after the operation, I asked him if he was coming again to talk to our friends.

"No," he said, "I'm going to come and play."

He played one set, sat out for two, then played again. He said he felt fine after the exercise and the psychological effect of being able to play tennis again without any ill effects, after those months of needing to take anginine to avoid chest pains, was tremendous. This was indeed a landmark in recovery.

Another was his change in attitude towards going to the surf. The previous summer, about six months before the attack which precipitated the bypass operation, he asked for a boogie-board for Christmas. A good surfer when young, he enjoyed body-surfing, but by the time that summer came he was evidently finding even a small surf too much for him. I bought him a boogie-board: he used it once. After that he would make excuses not to go to the surf. Sometimes after tennis I would suggest that we go to the beach: invariably the tennis had been as much as he could take that day and he would spend the afternoon resting and reading the paper. About four months after his bypass and several weeks after he began playing tennis again, as we drove home one hot day, I said, "We are mad. We should have gone to the beach instead of playing tennis."

"All right," he said. "Come on. Let's get changed and go now."

I could hardly believe my ears. He brought his boogie-board, I took my surfoplane, we picked up some lunch on the way, and he said: "I bet that surprised you."

It certainly had, and that was the first of many enjoyable times at the beach during the rest of the summer. By then he was sailing again, too, being sensible and not taking the boat out if the forecast wind was too strong for comfort or for us to manage together. In other words, he could do as much as his body — his muscles, back and general strength — would allow without any risk of pain.

Different people take different lengths of time to return to their normal activities. Some have greater limitations before their operation, some are older, some may have had minor complications such as a temperature or fluid in the lung while in hospital. A lot depends on the patient's attitude to recovery, too. If he or she is determined to make full use of the new lease of life given by the coronary bypass graft, then normal activity is likely to return more quickly than for someone who is overcautious.

A lot depends, too, upon the attitude of the patient's partner and family. If they encourage prolonged convalescence the patient may heed them and not do as much as could be done. If they encourage self-help then the patient will do more and more each day and will feel delighted that these things can be done. Looking back to the period in hospital and comparing it with the activities possible after a few weeks at home usually makes the patient feel full of the joy of living.

The return to normal life affects people in different ways. Some become more aware of the problems of others. Some seem to have personality changes. Andrew suddenly realised in early middle age that he was not immortal and became very religious. Bill, about forty, seemed to change from a young man to a middle-aged man, his wife said. Some people seem to become very demanding at home and quite difficult — but this may be the person's own personality traits emphasised by the experience of pain and the operation.

Some people do have an occasional recurrence of chest pain, which they notice is associated with stressful situations. Some people retire a few years early, spend more time in leisure activities, or take on less onerous positions with the same firm. Others change their occupation — a truck driver decided to try farming, for instance.

Exercise is very important for the human body. Although Australians are considered (or consider themselves) a healthy outdoor people, there are many whose idea of sport is to watch others perform. Many others in sedentary work drive from home to office, sit most of the day, then drive home and spend the evening sitting. The post-operative walking programme should be continued. If a person normally plays sport he or she should return to that sport as early as feasible after a bypass operation. If the person normally does not then walking every day is a good form of exercise. Or, with the new lease of life, the person may feel inclined to take up some form of sport.

Golfers who have bypass surgery can return to the golf course and play, after about seven weeks. One hears of people taking up golf after a bypass, never having played before, and becoming champions! Bowlers, tennis players, swimmers, whatever your sport, ask your cardiologist when you can resume playing; you will be surprised how soon it is possible.

One woman complained, four months after her

operation, that she was allowed only to play doubles in tennis, not the energetic singles she enjoyed! Another woman felt unable to play tennis at all for six or seven months. Another, who had not played tennis for many years, began again and now plays regularly.

One woman, who was a keen yoga exponent, was able once again to stand on her head only three months after surgery; she complained of some discomfort (but not chest pains) when she did this four times in succession! How many people can stand on their heads even once?

Brian's principal landmark for recovery was when he was able to resume jogging about ten weeks after his bypass.

The list goes on and on. Everyone with a positive attitude to recovery finds more and more activities are possible as the weeks and months after the operation cause the memory of the discomfort to fade into the background.

CHAPTER 15

"Join the Club"

At the first symphony concert we attended after my husband's operation, when he was still feeling his way a little, a long-time friend came over to us.

"I hear you had a bypass," he said. "Join the club."

He told us that he had undergone the operation nearly fifteen years earlier—he must have been one of the very early patients—and we had not known this. He looked the same, apart from growing older, of course, as when we first knew him more than thirty years ago. He told us how well he had been since his operation.

We kept meeting people who had been so much healthier and more active since their bypass operations: it was surprising how many people had benefited from this operation. (In Australia more than six thousand men and women each year now "join the club" and with a risk of less than two per cent.)

Our friend was speaking symbolically when he said, "Join the club," but there are, in fact, Open Heart Surgery clubs in Sydney, Canberra and other centres. Their members visit people recovering from bypass surgery in hospital and at home, discuss with them any problems they may have (general problems with which they may not want to worry their doctors), and are supportive to their families. They go even further and arrange outings, dinners, golf and bowls days. Some people like to continue an association with others who have shared this experience; some people, having gone through the drama and trauma, and then the excitement of a new lease of life, prefer to put that past behind them. As David said, "Forget about it and get back into life again." This is a sentiment with which my own husband agrees.

Seven months after his operation we attended an international conference in Perth, preceded by a professional meeting at Festival time in Adelaide where we also attended some of the Festival performances. This trip meant two weeks away from home, being out every night, being constantly with other people, and the long flight back to Sydney from Perth. My husband was able to enjoy it all without turning a hair. Two months later he had to attend another meeting in Adelaide. I let him go without me, and this was the first time for several years that I had felt confident that he would be all right without me as a watchdog. He also travelled interstate for one-day meetings a number of times. Whereas he had often come home exhausted in the past, these trips no longer worried him, so much so that if we had something planned for the evening he was quite happy to go out.

My husband now looks, feels and acts ten years younger than before he had the bypass, and he has recently agreed to take on a senior official position in an Australian professional organisation. He is planning an overseas tour with several work sessions, where he will give lectures and attend conferences in Europe, to begin on the first anniversary of his admission to

115

hospital for the bypass operation.

We are not taking risks. We are aware that it is possible, given the same set of circumstances, for another artery to block, causing chest pains or another coronary, so he is trying to keep his weight down, he is watching his diet, and avoiding situations which could cause abnormal stress, making sure that he has plenty of rest and plenty of exercise. For those to whom it may be relevant, let us add to the foregoing precautions: no smoking.

One of the greatest advantages of bypass surgery is the freedom from angina and the freedom from fear that exertion will result in chest pains.

People who have been advised that a coronary bypass, although not essential, would help their heart condition, on seeing the improved abilities of those who have had the operation usually decide to undergo it themselves.

Doreen, advised two years ago that a coronary artery graft would help her considerably, had been procrastinating until she saw how well my husband was after only a few weeks. She made arrangements, had the operation, and four months later was able to undertake a long trip overseas.

Recently, an acquaintance, Warren, told me that he played golf with two men, one of whom had undergone bypass surgery. The other player was trying to decide whether or not to have the operation and asked the first for information.

"I learnt a lot, too," said Warren. "And after that golfing-round conversation I think he was convinced of the benefits of the operation."

When I told my husband about this, his comment

was, "If the cardiologist advises and recommends it, I'd advise them to go ahead and have it. Every time."

And this seems to be the feeling generally expressed by those people who have needed and benefited from coronary bypass operations. When they say, "Join the club," it is a welcome to others to an extension of happy, healthy and productive living.

Appendix 1

AVOIDING A CORONARY

Here are a few dos and don'ts that could help avoid a coronary attack:

1. Don't become overweight. If you are overweight, try to reduce.

2. Be careful about your diet. Have your doctor arrange a blood test if you suspect the level of cholesterol in your blood is high.

3. Make sure you have regular exercise. Walk, jog or swim daily, or play one of the more strenuous games (golf, tennis, squash, etcetera) once a week. Remember that sport does not have to be competitive to be enjoyable; it might be of more benefit to you if you do not have the tension of being all out to win.

4. Avoid excessive cigarette smoking.

5. Be organised at work; do not be continually "chasing your tail". Delegate those things not absolutely necessary for you to do yourself to someone

capable. Try not to take work home; learn to relax when not at work.

6. Limit outside activities to those you feel are really worthwhile or that you really enjoy.

7. Have an annual medical check-up; it is not a luxury but a form of insurance.

Warning to families: If someone seems unable to sit down and relax for more than a brief period, and if, along with this, he or she seems to be talking more than usual and more quickly than is normal — as if there is not enough time to say all he or she has to say — insist that he or she go to a doctor for a check-up.

WHEN A CORONARY OCCURS

A sudden, deep chest pain that sometimes extends into the arm (usually the left one), accompanied by shock (the patient is pale and cold, yet sweats), indicates a coronary. All chest pains are not coronaries, but if it is sudden and severe, and especially if there are shock symptoms, ring your doctor immediately.

Keep the patient warm.

Do not let him or her walk around and do things. Insist that he or she sit or lie quietly until medical help can be obtained.

If the family doctor is unavailable, the receptionist will usually arrange to send another doctor or an ambulance. If not, call the ambulance yourself by phoning the Emergency number (000 in Australia).

When a "collapse" or a "heart attack" call is received it is given priority and the nearest ambulance is sent immediately, even if it has to be diverted from another, less urgent, call.

There are also special coronary care ambulances available, which can be contacted by phoning the Emergency number.

CORONARY-ARTERY BYPASS SURGERY UNITS

Brisbane:
   Prince Charles Hospital

Sydney:
   Royal North Shore Hospital
   Royal Prince Alfred Hospital
   Westmead Hospital
   St Vincent's Hospital
   Prince Henry Hospital
   Sydney Adventist Hospital

Melbourne:
   Alfred Hospital
   St Vincent's Hospital
   Royal Melbourne Hospital
   Epworth

Adelaide:
   Royal Adelaide Hospital

Perth:
   Royal Perth Hospital

DIET

Instructions regarding diet vary from patient to patient depending on the body chemistry and weight. In most cases it is not necessary to cook special foods; the diet suitable for the coronary sufferer is suitable for the whole family. It is a balanced diet and may even be more beneficial than the usual food pattern.

The following general points are aimed at keeping down both weight and the amount of animal fat in the diet, and are based on the recommendations of the dietitian at the Royal Prince Alfred Hospital, Sydney.

Avoid:

> Cream, ice-cream (unless made with skim-milk powder and oil), whole milk, butter, cheese
>
> Dripping, chicken fat, lard, solid frying oils
>
> Fat meats—rib and rolled roasts; porterhouse, blade or T-bone steak; pork and fat bacon; lamb loin and shoulder chops; sausages and prepared sausage; canned meats
>
> Mayonnaise, unless polyunsaturated (most commercial varieties are made with safflower oil and are all right)
>
> Pastry, steamed puddings, cakes
>
> Fried foods and casseroles, unless suitably prepared.

Eat sparingly:

> Foods that contain cholesterol: brains, liver, kidney, tripe, shellfish—once a week; egg yolks (whether as breakfast egg or in sauce or custard or in other cooking)—limit to two a week
>
> Foods that have a high carbohydrate content:

potatoes, rice, bread, pasta, cereals, sugar, alcohol

Safe foods:

Skim milk, skim-milk yoghurt, cottage cheese

Polyunsaturated margarine

Vegetable cooking oils: safflower, sunflower, soya bean, maize, cottonseed

Lean beef or lamb: topside or fillet roasts; round, rump or fillet steak; yearling steak; roast leg of lamb; grilled chump chops — three or four times a week

Veal: any cut — allowed fairly often, as it has so little fat

Chicken, turkey, rabbit, fish (including smoked and tinned) — no limit

Vegetables, except potatoes and sweet potatoes

Fat-free soups

Fat-free pickles and relishes

Salad dressings made with polyunsaturated vegetable oil

Homemade ice-cream made with skim-milk powder and oil

All fruit and fruit juices

Coffee, tea and cocoa made with skim milk

Remember:

Poultry and fish contain as much protein as equal quantities of meat.

Count calories when serving potatoes, cereals or pasta (1 cup potato = 1 cup rice = 1 cup pasta).

Sometimes a typical Italian meal — a small helping

of pasta plus lean meat, and a salad—can be served as a change. Use polyunsaturated oil or margarine in the cooking.

Herbs, mushrooms, onions, garlic or wine added to chicken, veal or rabbit give variety in flavour without affecting the food value of the meal.

Salads are vitamin-rich and provide variety.

Mixed platters of fresh fruit in season make an attractive, nutritious and non-fattening dessert.

Many good recipes will be found either in the National Heart Foundation's booklet "Planning Fat-Controlled Meals" or its book *Guide to Healthy Eating*.

EXERCISE

Exercises to be done at home should be sanctioned by the doctor and started when he or she advises. They range from standing up and sitting down again twice a day to doing thirteen press-ups a day; from walking 800 metres in fifteen minutes to walking one and a half kilometres in seventeen minutes (to be achieved, usually, by the twelfth week).

The National Heart Foundation offers booklets on exercise and the book *Guide to Exercise*.

HOBBIES, HANDICRAFTS AND HOME GAMES

While the patient is in hospital the occupational therapists will introduce and explain a handicraft, and inform the patient's relatives where equipment may be bought or hired for home use. It will usually be found that the equipment needed for the following suggestions is available at retail stores, stationers', artists' suppliers or hobby shops in most cities. The Occupational Therapists Associations in each state will also give information on where to purchase equipment.

The Department of Health in New South Wales has established the Consultative Council for the Physically Handicapped which, at the request of a doctor, will send an occupational therapist to help pensioners in their homes.

Suggestions:

> Painting and drawing (watercolours, oil-paintings or number-pictures; pencil, pen-and-ink, charcoal or pastel drawings)
> Small sculptures (wood, clay or plasticine) or moulds
> Knitting
> Crochet
> Basketwork
> Leatherwork
> Rug-making
> Lampshade-making
> Weaving (on small looms): table-mats, scarves, etcetera
> Artificial-flower-making (coloured paper, nylon, or plastic)
> Tapestry: pictures, cushion- and chair-covers, handbags
> Mosaics: trays, table-tops, dishes
> Toy-making (felt, rag or knitted)

Model-making: aeroplanes, boats, etcetera

Writing: articles, travel tales, short stories, memoirs, letters, radio or TV scripts, children's stories, educational or technical works, plays, novels

Music: listening to radio or records, reading the lives of musicians, or learning an instrument

Studying of all kinds: teach-yourself books, private tuition, tapes or records

Light gardening: pot-plants, bonsai, etcetera

Light carpentry

Training a bird or an animal: a budgerigar to talk; a puppy in obedience

Collecting: stamps or coins

Cataloguing: a collection, perhaps the colour-slides that have been waiting so long, or photographs that need arranging in an album

Bridge (inquire at your local bridge club about teachers)

Solo or other card-games (books available containing rules of play)

Chess, draughts, dominoes, solitaire, etcetera

Jigsaw puzzles

Crossword puzzles (in the daily papers, and in books of crossword puzzles)

Scrabble (small "travel" sets available that can be managed quite easily in bed).

Appendix 2

(Compiled by Jenny Mulherin)

BRITISH ASSOCIATIONS AND SERVICES FOR HEART AND CORONARY ADVICE, CARE AND REHABILITATION

In Britain, 6100 coronary-artery operations were performed in 1981. Bypass operations represent the fastest growing section of cardiac surgery, accounting for well over half of all surgery in the adult population.

Heart and coronary associations and services in Britain include the following:

1. The UK equivalent of the National Heart Foundation of Australia is the British Heart Foundation, 102 Gloucester Place, London W1H 4DH. This is a charitable organisation that aims to: encourage and finance research into cardiovascular disease and its prevention; inform doctors of advances in research, etcetera; inform the public about risk factors through the publication of the Heart Research series of pamphlets (titles include "Back to Normal" (heart attacks), "Recovery from a Stroke", "What is Angina?", "Smoking and Your Heart", "Heart Surgery for Adults"); and improve facilities for cardiac care. The British Heart Foundation does not generally offer practical help or advice to the public, except in the

form of pamphlets, but rather to NHS doctors, hospitals, etcetera.

2. The Chest, Heart and Stroke Association, Tavistock House North, Tavistock Square, London WC1H 9JE, another charitable organisation, can be helpful to the public by referring them to suitable volunteer organisations, but does not itself provide advice.

3. There are a number of voluntary organisations that help people who have undergone open heart surgery. Two are: Take Heart, c/o Mr George Morland, 55 Flaxpiece Road, Claycross, Chesterfield S54 9MD; and Heartline, 47 Kettering Road, Rothwell, Northampton. For information on organisations in other areas, contact the Chest, Heart and Stroke Association at the above address.

4. Rehabilitation units operate in various parts of Britain but referral to them is in the hands of a patient's doctor. In addition, places in these units are limited so there is a waiting list on the NHS. Rehabilitation problems can be discussed with your doctor who may advise you to contact one of the voluntary organisations that help with heart and coronary problems.

5. Coronary care ambulances operate in some parts of Britain and their use is being extended into country districts. They do not operate in London where the aim is to get the patient to hospital as quickly as possible. However, all ambulance crews are trained to deal with cardiac arrest, resuscitation, etcetera.

6. In cases where an ambulance is needed urgently,

the Emergency telephone number in Britain is 999.

Other information relevant to Britain:

1. Information on schemes for giving up smoking can be obtained from ASH, 27-35 Mortimer Street, London W1N 7RJ, or from the Chest, Heart and Stroke Association.

2. The recipe book *Cooking for Your Heart's Content* is available from the British Heart Foundation at the above address for £4.50 (including postage and packing) or as a paperback for £1.10 (including postage and packing).